THE 168 HOUR CAREGIVING WORK WEEK:

ACTIVITY QUICK GUIDE

Activity Ideas For:

- Alzheimer's Disease
- Lewy Body Dementia
- Frontal Lobe Dementia
- Vascular Dementia
- Parkinson's Disease
- Traumatic Brain Injury
- Huntington's Disease
- Stroke
- - and more

Carson and Monty

Disclaimer

This book is for informational purposes only and is not intended as medical advice, diagnosis, or treatment. Always seek advice from a qualified physician about medical concerns and do not disregard medical advice because of something you may read within this book. This book does not replace the need for diagnostic evaluation, ongoing physician care, and professional assessment of treatments. Every effort has been made to make this book as complete and helpful as possible. It is important, however, for this book to be used as a resource and idea-generating guide and not as an ultimate source for plan of care.

Activity Quick Guide

The 24/7 job of caregiving is stressful enough without struggling to figure out things for your loved one to do so they are not just staring out a window, nodding off throughout the day.

This book is designed as a quick guide for ideas to engage the one you care for. These are just starting points to get your creative juices flowing so you can design activities that your loved one can participate in and enjoy.

Throw away any pre-conceived notions you and others may have on how something should be done. There is no right or wrong way when it comes to activities. There is only what works for you and your loved one.

Table of Contents

Planning and Executing Activities

Millions of family caregivers struggle with getting their loved one to "do something". It is the same for staff and activity directors in various long-term care settings like nursing homes. The key to success is a two-part process:

1. Find a topic your loved one enjoys.

2. Create a new activity or modify an existing activity to allow your loved one to be successful regardless of their physical or cognitive limitations. Please remember it does not matter what others think about the activity, what matters is your loved one enjoys it and can do it.

A Topic They Enjoy

This refers to the idea that each person has a personal identity and history. When you are figuring out what their interests are, you must also remember the word CRANE. The word crane is a homonym – to some, it means a type of bird. To others, it means a piece of machinery used to lift objects.

If we look at gardening as an activity, we need to figure out what our loved one's definition of gardening is.

Is it going outside, cutting the grass, trimming the hedges, and weed whacking? Is it getting in the flowerbeds, planting flowers and vegetables, and tending to the garden on their hands and knees each day?

Allow Them to Be Successful

This concept considers the varying functional levels at which a person may be able to participate in any activity. Modifications might be needed either by using different steps or by using adaptive tools so your loved one can still enjoy the activity. Based on your loved one's functional level and abilities, some activities might be done as a group activity. This creates an opportunity for socialization, interaction, and conversation between you and your loved one.

Let's use gardening again. If your loved one enjoys getting in the flowerbeds, planting, and tending to the garden on their hands and knees each day, but can no longer get down in the garden to plant, a modification may be to use adaptive equipment to allow them to plant seeds while seated in their chair. The planted seeds can be placed in their room on the near a window, so they can water the seeds and watch them grow. Once the seeds sprout, they can then be planted outside with assistance from others.

Sensory Activities: Smell

Sensory stimulation uses everyday objects to arouse one or more of the five senses: hearing, sight, smell, taste, and touch with the goal of evoking positive feelings.

Smells are a great way to engage our loved one and help them on their way to a happy day. You can also use each of the smells below as a reminiscing tool or discussion starting point for a conversation about memories the smell reminds them of.

<u>Essential oils and Lotions</u>

- Place drops of essential oils on cotton balls and pass them around to identify scents.
- Place rubbing lotions on wash cloths and pass them around. Talk about what the smells remind you of.
- Squish wax with lavender in your hands. It's great for arthritis and helps relax and hydrate the hands.
- Small scented sachets can be used as well. Place a small piece of pillow/craft stuffing

on a small fabric square. Scent the stuffing with a few drops of essential oils such as lavender, mint, bergamot, or verbena on the small fabric squares. Tie the sachet with pretty ribbon.

- Place a few drops of essential oil in a diffuser or humidifier.
- Mix a few drops of an essential oil with an unscented lotion. Use the scented lotion for a gentle hand massage.
- Burn a candle scented with the desired essential oil.
- Put a scented candle into a glass jar and then place the jar on an electric cup warmer.

<u>Items in the Kitchen</u>

- Cut open fruit and let your loved one hold them, smell them, and maybe eat them.
- Place "homey" spices such as cinnamon, nutmeg, cumin, and oregano on a cotton ball. Place the cotton ball in a small plastic container and pass it around allowing everyone to enjoy the aroma.

- During fall and winter, keep cinnamon sticks, oranges slices, cloves, and maybe some apples in a pot with water on the stove. Heat as needed to activate the aroma.
- Juice oranges and lemons by rolling them, cutting them in half, and then squeezing the juice out. Enjoy the aroma.

<u>Baking and Smells</u>

- Make bread on certain days of the week, like Mondays.
- Bake cookies.
- Bake treats like Lemon cake, gingerbread men, strawberry cake, pies, and Bundt cakes.
- Bake seasonal recipes. For example, in October, you can enjoy the smells of the season by making pumpkin muffins, Crock-Pot veggie soup, or Crock-Pot apple cider.
- Cut an orange in half along the equator, cutting only the peel, and not the fruit. Stick your fingers between the peel and the fruit and pop the fruit out while keeping

the peel intact. Take the orange peel halves and use them as cupcake liners, pouring the cupcake batter into the orange peel cupcake liners.

- Brew coffee.

Seasonal Scents

- Around any holiday, focus on a scent associated with that holiday. For example: roses for Valentine's Day and pine for Christmas.

Garden Scents

- Place different herbs in small covered boxes. Each person picks a box to guess what smell is in the box and discusses what the smell reminds them of.
- Flowers. The same activity for herbs can be used for different flowers.
- Make fruit infused water by filling a pitcher to the top with ice and fruit. Fill the pitcher with cool water. Let sit for at least one hour. Poking holes in the fruit helps to

release the flavors faster. Some tasty and unique smelling flavors include: kiwi-orange, raspberry mint, strawberry basil, cucumber lemon, and blueberry lime.

- Create delicious herbal drinks by infusing lemonade with herbs from the garden. Try lavender, rosemary, elderflower, or watermelon-basil. Smell first, then sip.
- Do you have mint in your garden? Freeze whole mint leaves into ice cubes. You can also mince the herbs and pack them into an ice cube tray, until about ¾ full. Fill the tray with hot water and carefully place in the freezer.
- Create herb butter by pouring either extra-virgin olive oil or melted, unsalted butter over herbs. Cover the container lightly with plastic wrap and let freeze overnight.

Sensory Activities: Touch

Sensory stimulation uses everyday objects to arouse one or more of the five senses: hearing, sight, smell, taste and touch. The goal is to evoke positive feelings.

Here are some ideas for sensory activities using touch:

- Mix 1-part hair conditioner and 2-parts corn starch to create an extremely soft play dough.
- Make stress balls to squeeze and roll in hands. Using a funnel, place the stem inside the balloon. Pour flour into the balloon until it is almost completely full. Let out any extra air and tie the balloon.
- Make Silly Putty. Pour ½ cup of corn starch and ½ large package (1.55 oz.) of sugar-free gelatin into a bowl. Add 2 tablespoons of water and stir. Continue to add water until putty forms.
- Hand massage
- Foot massage

- Make your own bubble solution by mixing ½ cup of dishwashing liquid, 1 ½ cups of warm water, and 2 tablespoons of glycerin. Pop the bubbles as they float.
- Use a bubble machine. You can set the bubbles to shoot out quickly or slowly. Add food coloring to create rainbow bubbles!
- Sensory bags. Choose a variety of small, non-sharp objects (plastic toys, buttons, coins, pebbles, gems, glitter, beads, pearls, game pieces, rubber toys) and one shade of food coloring. Use a plastic zip-top sandwich bag and edge the three sides with duct tape. Open the zip side of the bag and pour in a clear gel, shaving cream, or sand until the bag is almost full. Add the objects and a couple of drops of food coloring. Squeeze out any remaining air and tape shut. Feel the objects through the bag.
- Foot or hand spa. Gather a plastic basin, towels, lotion, Epson salts or essential oils, and a nail file (optional - nail polish and nail polish remover). Soak your loved ones' feet or hands in the scented basin of warm

water. Remove appendages and dry with towels. Give a gentle massage with lotion. File nails as needed.

- Soap Making. Add 4 cups of grated, hypoallergenic soap, 2 tbsp. of hand cream, 3 tbsp. warm water, and ½ tsp essential oil into a mixing bowl. Cover your hands with lotion and use them to mix the ingredients. Shape the soap by hand or use molds to shape. Let harden.
- Different textures. Gather pieces of different fabric, such as: calico, velour, velvet, leather, fur, corduroy, lace, hemp, silk, wool, chiffon, etc. Lay a few fabrics at a time onto the participant's lap, allowing them to feel the fabric.
- Home made snow. Combine 3 cups of baking soda and ½ cup of white hair conditioner. Mold into a ball and store in a sealed, plastic bag in the fridge.
- What's in the bag? Place common, household items in an opaque bag (spoon, clothespin, brush, eraser, sock, key, spatula, etc.). The participant places their

hand in the bag to touch one item and
attempt to guess what it is.

Activities for Low Functioning Adults

- Flower arranging. Use a spaghetti strainer and fake flowers. Let your loved one arrange the flowers through the holes.
- Create a puzzle. Use magazine or printed pictures of kids or pets, cut them into 4 pieces or 5 pieces (or more depending on their skill level).
- Gather several small, plastic farm and jungle animals. Place them in a bucket of dirt. Give your loved one the bucket, a bowl of water, and a tooth brush. Have them clean the animals, "so the kids can play with them".
- Sort playing cards - first black and red and then by suit if they can.
- Sort poker chips.
- Sort baby socks.
- Fold the socks once they have been sorted.
- Fold towels so they can be put away.
- Clip coupons.
- Make a Galaxy bottle - Fill half of a plastic bottle with baby oil. Add glitter to the

bottle. Create dark blue water by adding food coloring to water. Pour the blue water into the bottle until the bottle is almost full. Place the cap onto the bottle and secure with tape. Shake and watch.

- Sensory and reminiscing boxes
  - Military service
  - Past occupations
  - Cooking
  - Jewelry box
  - School days
  - Childhood
- Photo albums
- Picture books
- Catalogues
- Try on scarves, hats, and jewelry.
- Color match using color folders and color paper. Have them put the color paper in the matching color folder.
- Sort buttons
- Doll therapy

Writing and Coloring Activities
- Writing
  - Address envelopes
  - Write name
- Coloring
  - Crayons or pencils
  - Use coloring books or print templates from internet

Writing and Coloring Activity Tips

- If your loved one has trouble holding a pen or pencil, wrap foam around the shaft of the pen to help your loved one's grip. You can try cutting a piece from a foam noodle used in a swimming pool to fit on the writing tool.
- Reduce glare and shadowing by positioning a chair and table so any natural light is behind them instead of coming at them from the front.
- To prevent shadows, place lamps on the opposite side of the hand being used.

- Locate the bottom edge of the lampshade just below eye level.
- Shiny paper can increase glare, so it's best to use matte paper when reading or writing.
- Use large-print crossword, word search or word scramble puzzles. See the R.O.S. *How Much Do You Know About* series of e-Books at Amazon or Barnes and Noble.
- A dry-erase board or tablet may also be used to practice writing.

** **Note:** Know the type of seating where your loved one is the most comfortable when they are writing, and, if possible, move them to that seat.

** **Note:** If your loved one is seated in wheelchair, recliner, or bed, provide a flat surface that fits in their lap to place paper on.

Purposeful Activities

As human beings, we all need to feel like we have a purpose, a reason to get out of bed, and a reason to get dressed for the day.

Here are some purposeful activities that your loved one can engage in to give them a sense of purpose:

- Shuck corn
- Tear lettuce and spinach for a salad
- Water plants
- Arrange flowers
- Set the table
- Sweep the floor
- Stuff envelopes
- Polish shoes
- Make the bed
- Organize receipts

You can tie into their past occupation or employer which they may have enjoyed working at during their lifetime. Here are some examples of how you can tie their past careers to an activity to engage them:

Business Owner

- If your loved always wanted to have a dressmaking business, validate those feelings and let them. Set up a desk with a typewriter, timesheets, ledgers, fabric, sketch pad, and mirror. Get them settled and oriented to their work station.
- Let them talk to you and others about the business and how to design clothes.

Accountant

- Save receipts. Have your loved one add them up. Separate food, toiletries, etc.
- Get your loved one a book to write some figures in a spreadsheet or on a ledger.
- Is there anything in the house to "inventory" such as napkins, silverware, towels? Record their findings.
- Let them dress for work each morning.
- Pack a lunch box.
- Set up a desk for them to work at.

Active Activities

Use it or lose it. There is always a way to keep your loved one active in some form or fashion if their doctor says it's okay. Modification is the key to allow your loved one to be successful.

Active activities can be broken into four areas that can help improve the quality of life for everyone. With new technology, access to videos through websites such as YouTube, Caregiving101.com, or streaming services such as Apple TV, it makes it easier than ever before to be active at home.

Aerobic Activities

Objectives of aerobic activities include: improving physical fitness and having positive effects on slowness, stiffness, and mood. Examples of aerobic activities include:

- Walking
  - with a family member, a friend, or a dog
  - on a treadmill or on a hike
  - in a city park or around the shopping mall
  - at a community garden or conservatory

- Swimming or water aerobics
  - at your gym or YMCA
- Riding a bike or cycling
  - around the neighborhood or on a stationary bike
- Dancing
  - at home with you, a family member, or a friend at a local dance hall, club, or ballet center
- Chair aerobics or Zumba
  - in your living room following along with a video or YouTube

Strengthening Activities

The objective of improving muscle strength is to make activities such as getting up from a chair or moving from room-to-room easier. Examples of strengthening activities include:

- Weights/resistance
  - free weight activities/exercises
  - elastic bands activities/exercises
  - body weight activities/exercises
- Yard work or gardening

Flexibility Activities

Objectives of stretching and flexibility activities include: improving range of motion which can affect posture and walking ability, reducing the risk of injury, and making everyday activities easier. Examples of flexibility activities include:

- Tai chi
- Gentle stretching
  - In your living room following along to a video
- Yoga, including chair yoga

Balance Activities

Balance activities can improve posture and stability. Preserving your loved one's ability to maintain their balance can help to reduce the likelihood of falling, potentially calm your loved one's fears of falling, and help them generally in performing daily tasks. Examples of balance activities include:

- Yoga, including chair yoga
- Tai chi
- At-home balance exercises using
  o A Wii
  o A balance ball or balance pillow

Active Games for Individuals or Groups

- Wii Bowling and other games
- Balloon volleyball. Use a balloon for a volleyball and a paddle made of something like a paper plate taped to a spatula, ruler, or paint stick (balloon ping pong).
- Whack a Balloon
- Corn hole
- Indoor Cornhole. Use tape on the floor to create the cornhole board
- Yard darts
- Indoor, seated soccer
- Use a balloon for a ball.
- Use tape or cardboard to create a goal
  o Indoor, seated bowling
  o Beach ball toss and basketball toss game

- Table hockey with dusters from the dollar store and balloon for pucks
- Hot potato with a whoopee cushion. When the music stops, the person with the whoopie cushion squeezes it.
- "Twisted Twister" - Spin the regular spinner. Instead of using feet and hands, toss bean bags at numbered circles.
- Fly Swat game - Using fly swatters, hit a balloon back and forth to each other. (balloon tennis)
- Pool noodle hockey - Have a group sit in a circle. Give everyone their own pool noodle. Throw a large plastic ball in the middle of the circle and have them pass it to each other.
- Use an old bed sheet as a parachute and place a few balloons or small balls on the sheet. Each person takes a side and lifts the sheet up and down to bounce the items inside.
- Backyard Games - place a ladder on the lawn and try to throw bean bags between the rungs or steps of the ladder.

- Backyard Games - place hula hoops onto the lawn at varying distances and try to throw bean bags inside of the hoops.
- Backyard Games - tape the ends of pool noodles together and use them as rings for ring toss or as a hoop for basketball.
- Use laundry baskets, empty dog bowls, or other household items for target toss games.
- Nerf guns and water guns are fun for outdoor target practice.

Entertainment, TV, and Movies

Television shows, movies, and various video sources are a great form of entertainment for your loved one. Whether it is following along with a game show, listening to classic radio programs, or enjoying a movie, there are plenty of entertainment options for you to plan into your loved one's day.

Movies and TV on cable, DVD, or streaming
- Watch movies and TV shows without violence or too much action. This can be upsetting to someone with dementia and they may not be able to distinguish between real life and TV life.
- Lawrence Welk programs
- Musicals
- History Channel

Game Shows
- Price is Right
- Wheel of Fortune
- Jeopardy
- Programs on the Game Show Channel

Internet Videos

- Animal YouTube videos
- Live webcams from zoos
- Eagle cams
- Live feeds to aquariums
- Laughing baby videos

Radio Programs and Music

- Old Time Radio shows
- Satellite radio stations
- Streaming music channels
- Cable TV music channels

Sports

- Watch favorite sports on TV.
- Listen to favorite sports on the radio.

Arts and Crafts

Arts and crafts are wonderful activities to engage your loved one with. Here are some tips and activity suggestions to try:

Craft Activity Tips

- Make sure that supplies are easily accessible.
- Empower your loved one by choosing an area of the home where they can most comfortably participate.
  - If at a table and in a wheelchair, make sure the wheelchair can fit under the table.
  - If in a recliner, use an activity surface that fits comfortably in their lap, and choose an activity that does not have too many pieces that may be hard to keep track of.
- Craft Boxes and materials
  - Place craft activity supplies in boxes clearly labeled with a broad-tipped black marker.
  - Group like items for activities together.

Craft Ideas

- Make greeting cards.
- Paint on canvas.
- Adult coloring books and colored pencils
- Make tie-blankets.
- Tear pieces of colored tissue paper and Mod Podge them onto a canvas board for a beautiful collage.
- Roll out a slab of air-dry clay and use cookie cutters to create ornaments.
- Use sharpie markers to draw designs onto wax paper. Tape the paper to a window for a stained-glass look.
- Paint pine cones and string together to create a seasonal garland.
- Mix equal parts liquid watercolors, white glue, and shaving cream to create a fun, 3D sensory paint.
- Hang up a piece of white paper outdoors. Use watercolors to paint various shapes and designs. Spray the drawings with a water bottle while they are still wet to create a wonderful mix of abstract art.

- Glue shells, buttons, or wood slices to a canvas to create different designs and shapes.
- Pour paint into an ice cube tray and place craft sticks into the middle of each paint cube. Freeze the ice cube tray until the paint is frozen. Pop the paint cubes out of the try, hold the craft sticks, and swirl the frozen paint cube across a sheet of paper to create a picture.
- String beads onto a leather or hemp cord to create bracelets and necklaces.
- Tie pieces of cloth around a piece of twine or a metal wreath frame to create rag garlands and rag wreaths.
- Use various washi tapes to cover vases, craft items, and stationery.
- Use puff paint to write words or create designs on Mason jars. Let dry and then use craft paint to cover the Mason jars for a colored 3D effect.
- Use different shape paper punches to create different colored shapes from paint chip samples. Glue on paper to create a

picture or string together to create a
garland.

- Paint a layer of Mod Podge onto a bottle.
  Wrap yarn from the bottom of the bottle
  all the way to the top. Use different colors
  to create a fun design.
- Create mandalas by placing various objects
  (buttons, shells, flowers, leaves, acorns,
  coins, etc.) in various circle designs.
- Lay pieces of lace on a canvas. Spray clear
  gloss paint over the lace and let dry.
  Remove the lace and paint the canvas with
  watercolors.
- Make edible paint by mixing either milk or
  sweet, evaporated milk and food coloring.
  Fun foods to paint and eat are
  marshmallows and popcorn!

Fun and Games

Any game that your loved one enjoyed throughout their life, can still be enjoyed. You may have to alter the game or use adaptive equipment to help your loved one depending on their cognitive and physical abilities.

Here are some suggestions for games you may enjoy together, with family, or a group of people.

- Card games
  - Poker
  - Crazy 8's
  - Go Fish
  - Poker
  - Euchre
  - Blackjack
  - Gin Rummy
- Dice Games
  - LCR (Left Right Center)
  - Yahtzee
  - Stuck in the Mud

- Puzzles
  - Choose puzzles with larger pieces. These are easier for your loved one to manipulate.
  - If your loved one becomes frustrated because puzzle pieces are sliding when being placed, try a magnetic puzzle and a metallic flat surface so the pieces stick when placed.
- Word games
- Easy trivia
- Magazine scavenger hunt
- Easy crossword puzzles
- Kick croquet
- Tic Tac Toe
- Oversized Jenga
- Dominoes
- Backyard Bowling
- Horseshoes
- Bottle Ring Toss
- Ladder Ball

Music Activities

Music is a wonderful tool to engage your loved one and change a mood. Below are multiple activities for you to try that involve music.

- Sing-a-long songs and movie musicals
- Pick a song beach ball. Write the name of a song in each colored section of the beach ball. When someone catches the ball, they have to sing or hum the song from the section of the ball facing them.
- Name That Tune
- Look up favorite musicians and songs on the internet.
- Have a kitchen band with pots and pans or utensils.
- Sing hymns.
- Reminisce about the music of childhood.
- Listen to old records.
- Exercise to music.
- Finish music lyrics.

- Learn different dance styles to popular music genres. Many of these can be adapted to be done in a chair.
- Write a new verse to a song.

Outings

No one wants to be stuck in a house all day. "Cabin fever" will eventually catch up to all of us. We need to get out even if it is just to step out on the back porch and let the sun shine on our face. Here are some examples of outings you and your loved one may enjoy:

- Scenic drives/mystery drives - Everyone's name gets put in a basket. Draw one name and ask the person, "Left, right, or straight?" After a few blocks, draw another name, etc. It's always fun to see where you end up.
- Cooking clubs
- Gardening classes/clubs
- Ballet performances
- Ice cream socials
- Events at the historical society or veteran's memorial or children's museum
- Farmers market
- Flea markets
- Aquariums and zoos
- Restaurants

- Apple orchards
- Bowling
- Going to a park
- Having a picnic
- Shopping
- Art museums
- A live show, play, musical, or choir performance
- Going to a library
- Dinner outings
- High school plays and musicals
- Animal shelters
- Movie theater
- Gardens and conservatories
- University campuses
- Book stores

Evening Activities

Evenings are a time to engage your loved one in activities that are calming, for it is close to bedtime.

Here are some activities to consider for the evening hours:

- Sorting
- Folding
- Aromatherapy
- Deep breathing exercises
- Prayer
- Petting the dog or cat
- Sitting in the rocking chair
- Reminiscing boxes
- Picture books
- Short stories
- Guided relaxation
- Reading
- Listening to music
- Taking a bath

Reading Activities

Reading or having a book read to us is something most of us have done and enjoyed throughout our lives. Below are some ideas and tips for reading activities to use with your loved one:

Reading Activity Tips

- Large-print books are available at most bookstores and libraries.
- Read to your loved one or take turns reading to each other.
- Listen to audio tapes and books on CD borrowed from your local library, or from the free Talking Books program sponsored by the National Library Service.
- If your loved one prefers reading to listening, many new mobile devices such as iPads, Kindles, and Nooks all have options to increase the font size and adjust the color contrast.

Book Suggestions

- The Secret Garden
- Little Women
- Treasures from Grandmas Attic
- Saving Simon
- The Commonwealth of Thieves
- The Mormon Murders
- The Choice, by Nicholas Sparks
- The Girl on the Train, by Paula Hawkins
- All the Light We Cannot See, by Anthony Doerr
- Chicken Soup for the Soul: Older & Wiser: Stories of Inspiration, Humor and Wisdom about Life at a Certain Age, by Jack Canfield and Mark Victor Hansen
- The Murder House, by James Patterson
- Blue: A Novel, by Danielle Steel
- Tale of two Cities
- Great Gatsby
- 1984
- Pride and Prejudice
- Of Mice and Men
- A Man Called Ove by Fredrik Backman

- The Art of Racing in the Rain by Garth Stein
- The Cherry Harvest by Lucy Sanna
- Cold Sassy Tree by Olive Ann Burns
- Dewey: The Small-Town Library Cat by Vicki Myron
- Fried Green Tomatoes at the Whistle Stop Café by Fannie Flagg
- The Musical Comedy Murders of 1940 by John Bishop
- Hometown Tales: Recollections of Kindness, Peace and Joy by Philip Gulley
- Teacher Man: A Memoir (The Frank McCourt Memoirs) by Frank McCourt
- Anything by Phyllis Diller, Erma Bombeck, or Jerry Apps

Resources

With over 250 activity ideas to get you started, this book is just one tool available to caregivers who struggle to get their loved ones to stay active and live the highest quality of life possible.

There are thousands of websites, books, support groups and companies here to support family caregivers around the world.

There is no right or wrong answer when it comes to engaging your loved one. The key is to make the effort and be ready to adapt all activities to your loved one's abilities.

We know that caregiving is a struggle. Stay strong and never give up.